Inès Bertille Koffi

Interjections in Ivorian

Inès Bertille Koffi

Interjections in Ivorian

Oh ! Hein ? Yako !

ScienciaScripts

Imprint
Any brand names and product names mentioned in this book are subject to trademark, brand or patent protection and are trademarks or registered trademarks of their respective holders. The use of brand names, product names, common names, trade names, product descriptions etc. even without a particular marking in this work is in no way to be construed to mean that such names may be regarded as unrestricted in respect of trademark and brand protection legislation and could thus be used by anyone.

Cover image: www.ingimage.com

This book is a translation from the original published under ISBN 978-3-639-62794-7.

Publisher:
Sciencia Scripts
is a trademark of
Dodo Books Indian Ocean Ltd. and OmniScriptum S.R.L publishing group

120 High Road, East Finchley, London, N2 9ED, United Kingdom
Str. Armeneasca 28/1, office 1, Chisinau MD-2012, Republic of Moldova, Europe
Printed at: see last page
ISBN: 978-620-8-16543-7

Contents

Interjections among Ivorian German students

Hein? Eh! Yako!

To my father

THANKSGIVING

I would like to take this opportunity to thank those who have supported me with their expertise, patience and encouragement during the writing of this thesis.

First of all, I would like to thank my supervisor, Professor Abo Justin KOUAME, who reviewed this Master's thesis and supported me throughout the entire process.

I would also like to thank Dr Dizo Austenne LOGBO, who gave me a lot of attention, advice and help. My sincere thanks also go to Mrs Maria Rauscher, whose advice really helped me to make progress with my research work. I am also grateful to my parents and friends for their financial and moral support.

Last but not least, I would like to thank all the participants in my surveys, especially Yala Kamanro, whose availability made a major contribution to the outcome of this master's thesis.

Introduction

This includes, in order, the presentation of our research topic, the motivation for choosing this topic, the problem, the hypotheses, the aim of the work, the critical state of research on the topic, the methodological procedure and the structure of the work.

0.1 General information on the topic

Interest in the German language has obviously spread throughout the world over the course of time. In Africa in particular, this language is learnt in schools and studied at universities. According to "Deutsche Welle" (DW), around 1.6 million of the 15.4 million German learners in 2020 came from Africa.[1]

Cote d'Ivoire is notable among the African countries that emphasise learning German. German has been learnt as a foreign language in this country since 1958[2] . It should be noted that Ivorian pupils learning German are mainly taught the basic principles of the language (linguistic knowledgc). At Ivorian universities, on the other hand, particular emphasis is placed on language competence (language skills). This means that students or students of German studies should be able to communicate in German. However, it has been found that these students often come up against rules when speaking that make it difficult to understand what they are saying.

One of the most common errors in communication is the incorrect use of interjections. This observation leads us to investigate the linguistic features underlying this incorrect use of interjections by 1st year German students. With this in mind, we formulate our research as follows: **Incorrect use of the**

Interjections in the conversation of 1st year German students (20212022) at the University of Felix I l()uph()uc˙ t-Boigny.

How did we come to choose this topic? The answer to this question can be found in the following section.

0.2 Motivation for choosing the topic

The interest in this topic arose from a remark. Indeed, in our academic experience at the University of Felix I loiiplioinel-Boigiiy, we have noticed that German students, especially first-year students, rarely refer to German interjections when talking to each other.

In order to express their feelings, students tend to use their own interjections in their own languages. These are, for example, interjections from their mother tongues (local languages in this case) or even interjections from French (the official language of the country). This inappropriate use occurs more and more frequently in the languages of the people concerned and has aroused our curiosity.

The need to identify and linguistically explain this incorrect use of interjections by 1st year German students is therefore of great interest to us. In addition, this study will be of benefit to academia as it will reveal further difficulties that students of German face

---

[1]Deutsche Welle: *Number of German learners in Africa*, online at: https://amp-dw.com/de/afrika-deutsch-als-trendsprache/a-54465700 last accessed on 30/01/2023 at 12:25.

[2] Cf. Augustin Agnimel, SESS *: L'enseignement de I'allemand dans les lycees et colleges de Cote d'Ivoire : Etude critique des methodes utiliseespour l 'enseignement de la langue et des contenusproposes en civilisation dans les manuels (1958-1992).* Doctoral thesis, supervised by Prof Jean Moes, Metz, 1994, p.14.

when using the German language. Now we can ask how this incorrect use can be challenged?

0.3 On the problems of the work

The first-year German students at the University of Felix Houpho^t-Boigny hardly ever use German interjections when communicating in German. This fact leads us to look for the linguistic features underlying this use. The fundamental problem that arises from our research topic is the following:

What are the psycholinguistic characteristics related to the incorrect use of interjections in 1st year German students at the University of Felix I loiiplioinel-Boigiiy?

In order to find an answer to this question, secondary questions are also asked:

- What semantic references do the interjections used by the first-year students contain?
- How can the interjections used be understood contextually?

Now we come to the hypotheses of the work.

0.4 About the hypotheses of the work

The hypotheses of our research are divided into main hypotheses and secondary hypotheses.

That is our hypothesis:

- First-year students at the University of Felix Houpho^t-Boigny use incorrect interjections in German.

Then there are the secondary hypotheses:

- German students are probably influenced by their mother tongue and culture in their use of interjections.
- The need to be understood leads to a mixing of interjections.

The objectives of this work are emphasised below.

0.5 Aim of the work

The main aim of this work is to raise awareness of the presence of German interjections among students of German studies. This results in secondary objectives, including

To sensitise lecturers to organise lessons in which students will learn German interjections.

To keep the interest of German students in the German language high.

After the objective, the critical research status of the work is discussed.

0.6 The critical state of research

Authors and linguists have dealt with the topic of "dealing with interjections". The main aim here is to summarise and assess some of the points of view that have been discussed in interjection research.

Firstly, Chaiqin Yang should be mentioned. The author wrote his doctoral thesis at the Albert Ludwig University in 2001, in which he compared German and Chinese interjections. In contrast to other German linguists, Chaiquin wanted to achieve monosyllabic languages in terms of interjection. This study thus reveals the shortcomings of German linguistics, which for a long time failed to provide a concrete answer to the question of the function of interjections. He wrote the following: " *While this question still remains distinct in linguistics, interjections in Chinese behave both as words and as sentences (...)* 3"

Although this analysis is enriching for us insofar as the author has analysed German interjections and opened up the study in monosyllabic languages, it is noticeable that this study was limited to a comparison. For our part, instead of a comparison, we want to compare the use of German interjections by Ivorian students of German.

In her book *"Interjection and Onomatopoeia" in Polish*[3] [4] , Nathalie Kosch analyses the role of interjections in today's electronic communication. The author describes interjections as a means of linguistic oeconomy, especially for young people. Nathalie Kosch has indeed managed to emphasise the contribution of the use of interjections in electronic communication. However, this originality does not end a broader research on the topic. Unlike the author, who has harmonised interjections and electronic communication, our analysis puts together Ivorian German students and German interjections.

In 2018, the topic of interjections was also addressed by Pierre Halte. In his article *"positionnement syntaxique des interjections et des ëmoticones: modalisation, portee, vise<e "5 ,* attention was drawn to interjections in written utterances. Our study, on the other hand, deals with a different aspect of the topic, i.e. the incorrect use of interjections in German, this time at both the oral and the written level.

Then comes Daniel Gutzmann. As a specialist in expressive languages, the German linguist wrote a book entitled *"Linguistik der Expressivitat "6* in 2019. In this book, he focuses on linguistic expressions that express emotions. Among these, Gutzmann emphasises interjections. This work focusses on interjections as a linguistic means of expressing emotions and is therefore partly helpful in the study, as it investigates the use of interjections in the student environment.

Also in 2019, Amel Fraisse and Patrick Paroubek emphasised another characteristic of interjections in their article " *les interjections pour dëtecter les emotions* "[5 6 7] . They described interjections as "signs of subjectivity". As with Daniel Gutzmann, this study therefore focusses on the nature of interjections. The aforementioned works seem important for the present research because the authors have identified such an important feature of interjections. This gives us further insight into the topic, even though the main focus of our research is to guide German students towards an appropriate use of interjections in the language of study.

---

[3]Y. Chaiqin*: Interjections and onomatopoeias in language comparison: German versus Chinese.* Doctoral thesis, supervised by Prof. Dr Ulrich Rebstock, Freiburg, 2001, p.174.

[4] K. Nathalie: *Interjections and onomatopoeias in Polish: An investigation of everyday use in the age of electronic communication*, Vienna, 2015, pp. 23- 24.

[5] H. Pierre : *Positionnement syntaxique des interjections et des emoticones : modalisation, portee, visee*, in "cahiers de praxematiques", 2018, online at https//shs.hal.science/halshs-01803669, last accessed on 11.07.2023, at 23 :13.

[6] D. Gutzmann: *Linguistik der Expressivitat*, University of Cologne: Institute for German Language and Literature I, 2015, p. 79.

[7] F. Amel / P. Patrick: *Les interjections pour detecter les emotions,* Caen, 2015, online at hhtps://hal.science/hal-01617186, last accessed on 29/03/2023 at 21:04.

In 2020, Johann Faust dealt with the topic of interjections in his book *"Funktionsanalyse des Lexems "krass" als Interjektion der Jugendsprache"*[8] . More specifically, this thesis analysed the function of the lexeme "krass" as a youth language phenomenon. Faust was thus content to emphasise the use of a lexeme. In this study, we do not follow the same line as the author. We want to analyse the incorrect use of several interjections.

All of these authors have dealt with the topic of interjection from different perspectives. With regard to this master's thesis, the emphasis will be placed on the incorrect use of interjections by first-year German students, more specifically those at the University of Felix Houpho^t-Boigny. This study thus opens up a new field of analysis.

0.7 Corpus, methodological procedure and structure of the work

In order to understand the linguistic features based on the incorrect use of interjections in the speech of 1st year German students at the University of Felix Houpho^t-Boigny, questionnaires were given to the students concerned. The choice of this corpus can be explained by the fact that it allows us to highlight the interjections used by the students in their conversations.

Our method therefore consists of analysing the meaning of each interjection used by the students, also stating its origin and, of course, justifying its use in the conversation of German students. To do this, we have adopted a theoretical approach. Thc thcory on which this work is based was conceived by the English philosopher Paul Grice.

In order to carry out this investigation well, the work is divided into two parts, namely a theoretical part and a practical part. The first part of this work will be concerned with a general definition of the terms "interjection" and "interference". To do this, we will use various definitional approaches. The types of interjection in the German language will also be dealt with here, as this is the subject of our study. We will then introduce a theory, namely Grice's theory, which will be of crucial importance for the second part of the work. The second part, the practical part of our work, is based on the use of German interjections in the speech of German students. Interjections from our collected corpus are used for the analysis.

[8] F. Johann: *Functional analysis of the lexeme "krass" as an interjection of youth language,* Munchen: GRIN Verlag, 2020, online at https://www.grin.com/document/,letzter Accessed on 02/07/2023 at 21:00.

PART I

THEORETICAL PART OF THE WORK

1. explanation of core concepts of the topic and overview of linguistic theory in connection with the work

In this part of our work, terms are scrutinised and explored, with particular attention paid to the terms "interjection" and "interference". The theory relevant to this work, Grice's theory, is then discussed.

1.1 General information on the term "interjection"

Before we come to the clarification of the term, let's take a look at the following text:
aha the Germans **ei** the Germans **hurray** the Germans **pfui** the Germans **ach** the Germans **nanu** the Germans **oho** the Germans **hm** the Germans **no** the Germans **yes yes** the Germans

This text was taken from the book "*Beispiele zur deutschen* Grammatik"[9] by Rudolf Otto Wiemer. Looking at the words in bold, you can already see that they are not here by chance. This means, for example, that the author is feeling joy, resignation or even surprise. These words are therefore called "interjections".

The term was borrowed from the French *interjection,* the English *interjection* and the German *interjection* in the 18th century from Latin and comes from *interiercio* (which means interjection, interjection), verbal noun of *intericere* and means to throw in between[10] . According to the Duden dictionary, the term "interjection" is defined more precisely as a *syntactically often isolated word-like sound formation that expresses feelings or requests or imitates sounds[11]* . In other words, interjections are word types that are almost different from ordinary words and are used to communicate feelings such as (joy, pain, surprise, request, etc.).

Goddard Cliff points out an important criterion according to which interjections can in any case be regarded as a clearly linguistic phenomenon. From a semiotic point of view, Goddard describes interjections as expressively orientated linguistic expressions. In this sense, they differ from other word classes. He formulates it more clearly with the following words:

From a semiotic point of view, interjection have an expressive function rather than the representational or symbolic function characteristic of ordinary words and sentence. Someone who utters Ugh! or wow! for example, may be expressing. Something like an immediate feeling of disgust or surprise/admiration, but they are not describing their feelings as someone can do by saying I'm disgusted or that's amazing in a simple formulation, interjections show rather than say.[12]

[9] W. Otto Rudolf: *Beispiele zur deutschen Grammatik (schritte neunzehn)*, Berlin: Wolfgang Fietkau Verlag, 1971, online at https://www.stichter.com/show/interkulturelles-lernen/episode:interkulturelles-lernen-gedicht-empfmdungsworter- von-rudolf-otto-wiemer-62035764, last accessed on 29 March 2023 at 22:02.

[10] Cf. Duden: *Etymologisches Worterbuch des Deutschen*, Berlin: Akademie Verlag GmbH, 1993, p.587.

[11] Duden: *Deutsches Universalworterbuch A-Z*, Mannheim: Duden Verlag, 1996, S.773.

[12] C. Goddard: *Interjections and emotions (with special reference to "surprise "and "disgust"),* Queensland, 2014, p.4: *"From a semiotic perspective, interjections have an expressive function rather than the representational or symbolic*

From this quote it can be seen that interjections have a communicative effect. In contrast to ordinary words (nouns, verbs, adjectives...), interjections are purely expressive expressions. Another important
The point is that interjections allow you to strongly express the human feelings and sensations of a dialogue partner. You could even say that they are spontaneous utterances that allow you to briefly express what you would otherwise have taken a long time to say.
Described as a language-specific phenomenon, interjections are available to people as a form of expression just like the usual words. To better understand what has been said, let us imagine the following illustration:

Figure 1 : *Expression of pain through a sentence and through a Interjection*

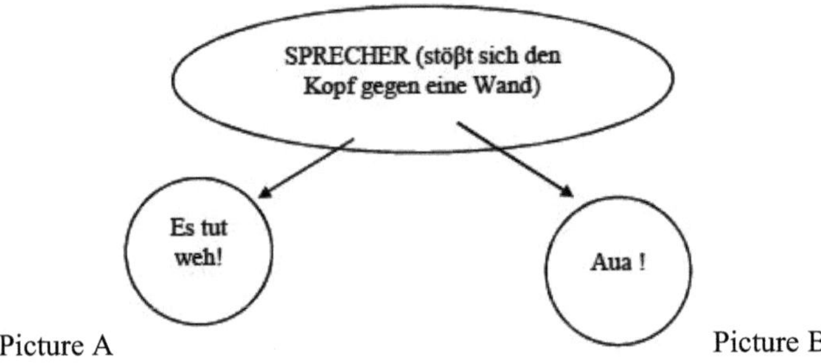

From this sentence it is clear that the speaker expresses a pain that the speaker has hurt his head.

Source: illustrated by me I.B. Koffi.

Two different situations are shown here. In picture A, someone is expressing pain. The statement "*it hurts*" makes it very clear to the speaker. In picture B, on the other hand, the speaker uses the interjection *"aua"*, which also expresses pain. Without a sentence, the speaker will realise that the other person is feeling pain. With an interjection, the feeling communicated by the speaker becomes clearer than with a sentence.
Goddard also makes a semantic distinction between volitional, emotive and cognitive interjections[13] . Volitional interjections are imperative expressions that are used to ask someone to do something. Emotive interjections are interjections whose main purpose is to express feelings in an emotional sense such as disgust, fear and anger, while cognitive interjections are used to express feelings related to cognition.
But how can the meaning of an interjection be recognised?

1.1.1 The meaning of the interjection

While it is possible to clearly determine the meaning of other types of words when

function that characterises ordinary words and sentences. For example, someone who says "Ipill'. " or "wow!" may be expressing something like an immediate feeling of disgust or surprise/admiration, but they are not describing their feelings in the way that someone who says "I'm disgusted" or "that's amazing" can do. Simply put, interjections show rather than tell. Translated by me, I.B. Koffi.

[13] Cf. ibid, p.5

they are used in a sentence, this is not the case with interjections. The meaning of an interjection depends heavily on certain parameters. For example, its meaning can be identified in connection with tonality. Konrad Ehlich identifies five tone patterns through interjection, namely falling, rising, level, falling-rising and rising-falling tonality[14] . Depending on the tone pattern, an interjection can therefore have different meanings. For example, the interjection *"oh"* in French can express pain, joy or surprise depending on the tone pattern. The English interjection *"hey"* also has different meanings depending on the intonation. On the one hand, it can express surprise and, on the other hand, it can express a huff. The same applies to the German interjection *"hm"*, which corresponds to different feelings. These are doubt, deliberation and agreement.

It is not only the tonality that helps to describe an interjection in linguistic action, but also the context in which it is used. To illustrate this, let's take this example:

Let's imagine two best friends who meet up again after several years. One of them tells you that she has just had a baby. The other, delighted and surprised at the same time, might say "*oh! What a surprise!"* If the other friend tells her that she has been ill for a long time, her friend could also say *"oh*!" with a different tone of voice. This time, however, to express empathy. So the same interjection was used in different contexts and with different tonalities to express different feelings. One obvious thing is that the communication partners are well aware of the meaning of the interjections used.

As we have seen, the meaning of an interjection is to a certain extent linked to pragmatics. In addition to the communicative function of interjections, in the next chapter we will discuss the subgroups into which they are categorised. We will do this using our own examples.

1.1.2 Categories of interjections

There are a large number of interjection variants, which can be categorised into 9 subtypes. These subtypes can be found in the online dictionary[15] :

Firstly, we have the words of speech, which fulfil a communicative function. They occur in human conversations and help to express concise intentions. For example, we have *"okay"* from English, "*ah"* and *"na ja"* from German, etc.

For example: (classmates chatting during the break)

Student 1: *We have a lot of work to do, we have an exam tomorrow.*

Schuler 2: ***well...***

In addition, the greeters must also be categorised. Like the first type of interjection, this type of interjection also fulfils a communicative function. The special feature, however, is that they are only used for greetings and farewells. Examples include words such as "*hallo"* from German, "*bye"* from English or "*tchao"* in French and "*tschau"* in German, as a version of the Latin word "*ciao"*.

The third category is called request words, which are also called appeal interjections. They are used to express urgent requests, such as "*chut"* in French, "*shh*" in English

[14] E. Konrad: *Interjektionen,* Tubingen: Max Niemeyer Verlag, 1986, p. 83.

[15] Interjection types, online at Wortwuchs.net/grammatik/interjection, last accessed on 20/08/2022, at 9:19.

and *"pst"* in German.

For example: (Children are in the classroom chatting during the lesson)

Teacher: ***shh!!!*** *(*instead of quiet please)

The so-called inflectives are a special form of interjections and are regarded as comic language. They are usually verb forms without a personal ending and are used to indicate the actions of a person or object in comics, such as *"boing"* for a muffled echoing sound, or *"klang"* for musical noises.

Delay sounds are interjections used in conversation to fill a pause in speech, e.g. *"hm"* from German, also common in French and English. For example: (schoolmates are planning to go to the cinema)

Schuler A: *Do you think Markus will come with you?*

Schuler B*:* ***hm,*** *I don't think so.*

Still called symptom interjections, the sensory words express the speaker's emotional affects and physical sensations such as pain, pity or disgust. With reference to Goddard, they can also be called emotive interjections. The following interjections belong to the symptom interjections: *"aua"* from German and *"aie"* from French for the expression of pain.

In addition to all these types of interjections, we have onomatopoeias used to imitate sounds and natural noises, for example animal noises such as *"cocorico"* from French and "*kuckuck*", which refers to the cockcrow and cuckoo sound.

Finally, the "words of other parts of speech" should be mentioned. These interjections are similar to the commonly known words, but their meanings in their use have nothing to do with the words as we know them, e.g. "*oh my God!*". You know that God is a term that stands for a higher being, but when you say *"oh my God"*, it can express great astonishment.

As we have just seen, there are different types of interjections, each of which has a specific function. These interjections can be found in all languages, even if they differ from language to language. In German in particular, there is a different classification of interjections that is well known even in the academic field. In order to better elaborate our analysis in the practical phase of the work, we will now look at the interjections of the German language.

1.1.3 On German interjections

After a general overview of the term "interjection", this chapter focuses on the interjections of the German language. Firstly, we look at their nature in the German language system, then we classify them. In addition, we show their function in each case.

1.1.3.1 Interjection as a particle

Also known as exclamations, interjections are categorised as particles in the German language system[16] . These are unchangeable words.

Unchangeable words are words that can neither be declined nor conjugated. In addition to interjections, this also includes adverbs, prepositions and conjunctions.

[16] Cf. Lubke Diethard: *Schulgrammatik Deutsch: Vom Beispiel zur Regel*, Berlin: Corneseln Verlag, 1999, p. 171.

These word classes cannot be changed in their use. In contrast to them, there are other word types that can be changed, namely nouns, articles, adjectives, pronouns, numerals and verbs. This can look like this:

Figure 2: *Parts of speech in the German language system*

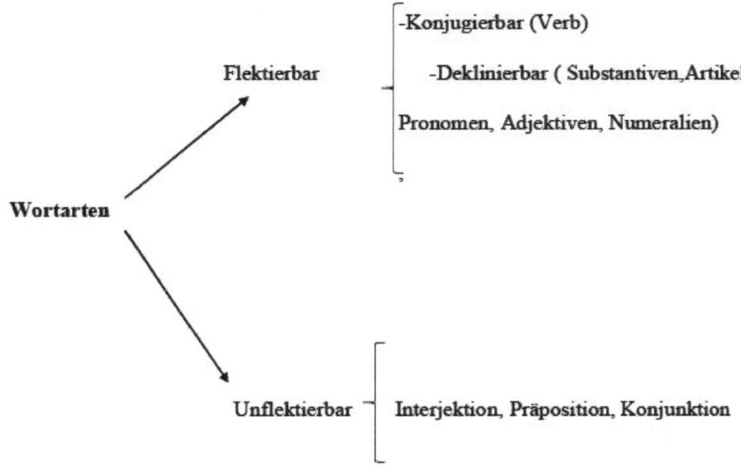

Word types
Inflectable
-Conjugable (verb)
-Declinable (nouns,articles
pronouns, adjectives, numerals)
Inflexible Interjection, preposition, conjunction
Source: illustrated by me I.B. Koffi.

This diagram shows the different word classes in the German language. Two categories appear from this. In the first category, only one word class is subject to conjugation, another word class includes declinable words, while other words in the second category can neither be conjugated nor declined, including interjections. The following sentences are examples:

Example 1: Go: Ali goes to school > The verb "gehen" is conjugated here and is changed from its original form.

Example 2: On: John buys a carThe article "on" becomes "a" in the Accusative.

Example 3: She has seen the child. She has seen the children > The noun "child" becomes "children" in the plural.

Example 4: Already: The beautiful lady there is called AndjibiThe adjective "already" becomes "schone" in the accusative.

Example 5: That: I say that I have seen him.

Example 6: From: Gerard's father is coming.

Example 7: Hurray: hurray! I've made it!

Source: Illustrated by me I.B. Koffi.

In example 5 there is a conjunction "*dass*", in example 6 there is the preposition *"von"* and in the last example there is an interjection *"hurra"*. In these examples, as you can see, the underlined words cannot be changed. Why are these word classes (conjunction, preposition, interjection) assigned to particles in the German language system?

In addition, interjections are particularly regarded as independent words. Used alone in a sentence, they are easily understood, e.g.

Example 1***: au!***

Example 2***: brr***

Source: Illustrated by me I.B. Koffi.

The interjections "*aua*" and "*brr*" indicate "pain" on the one hand and "disgust" on the other. When using these interjections, no further sentence elements are needed to make the meaning of both expressions visible. However, it would be pointless if we simply threw the word "tanze" into a sentence without adding anything. If another word is then added, e.g. a pronoun, a meaningful action would certainly result, as the following illustration shows:

Figure 3: *Meaningless and meaningful actions*

Ouch dance

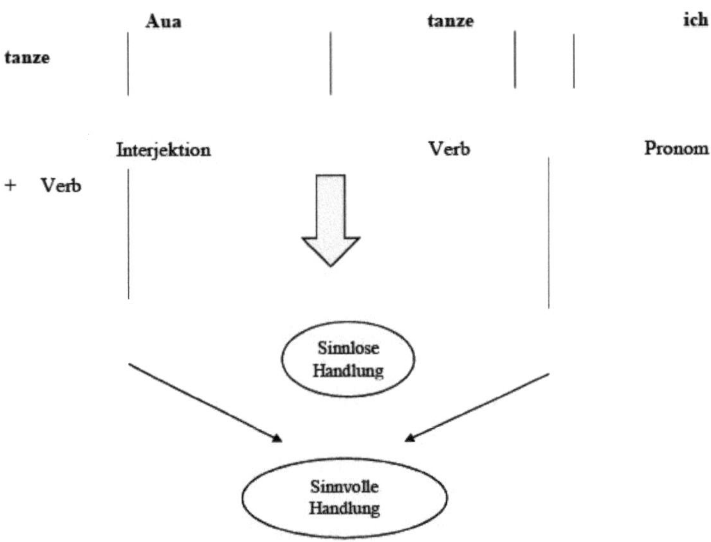

Source: Illustrated by me I.B. Koffi.

Once again, we see how interjections differ from other words. Interjections from German can also be easily differentiated into two categories. The next section consists of naming them.

1.1.3.2 Classification of German interjections

German interjections can be divided into two different groups: primary interjections and secondary interjections .[17]

1.1.3.2.1 What is primary interjection?

Primary interjections are called primaries because they already existed; they reflect natural sounds that were produced by humans. These interjections include sensory words and onomatopoeias. In general, single words are also regarded as primary interjections (aua, pfui, tja, ach). The primary interjections are not derived from any other word or word type.

Sensation words are actually used by language users without them realising that it is an interjection. They are feelings that are emphasised, things that do not require learning as they are linked to instincts. Although they imitate sounds, onomatopoeias still belong to this class because their production is linked to the acoustic phenomenon. In other words, onomatopoeias are produced by natural sounds.[18]

Figure 4: *Characteristics of the primary interjection*

Primary interjectio ns

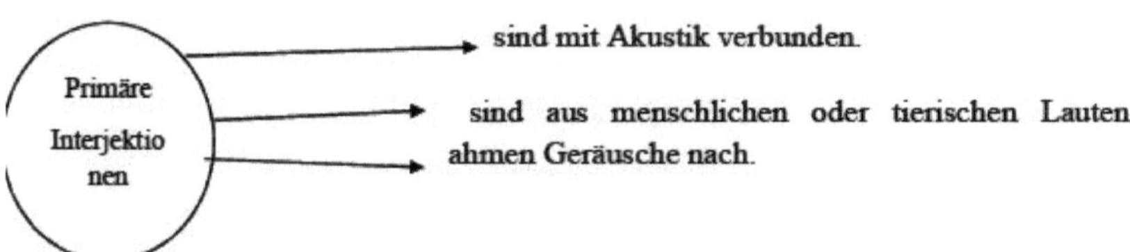

are connected with acoustics.

are made of human or animal sounds imitating noises.

Source: illustrated by me I.B. Koffi.

In addition to primary interjections, there are secondary interjections.

1.1.3.2.2 What does secondary interjection mean?

Emotional expressions that consist of words are organised into secondary interjections. Secondary interjections are, so to speak, nominal phrases such as *"oh God!", "good heavens"*, to express a surprise, something that was not expected. Ehlich says the following about the topic:

Especially expressions from the religious sphere, vocatives "vaporised" into formulas in which a deity is invoked or expressions from other taboo areas, especially scatological and genital expressions (merde!, fuck!) are used for this purpose[19]

These groups of words therefore come from the vocabulary of a particular language, but do not retain the same meaning when thrown into the sentence:

[17] Ehlich Konrad quoted by FOUAD Lobna: *The interjections in German and Arabic from a functional-pragmatic point of view*, Cairo, 2019, p.267

[18] Cf. FOUAD, Lobna: *The interjections in German and Arabic from a functional-pragmatic point of view*, Cairo, 2019, p.267.

[19] Ehlich Konrad quoted by F. Lobna: *Die Interjektionen im Deutschen und Arabischen aus funktional-pragmatische Sicht*, Universitat Helwan in Kairo, 2019, p.270.

You dear good one (That's very annoying.)
Oh dear! (I did something wrong.)
Exactly! (That's exactly what I mean.)
Good heavens! (this must not be true.)
Man oh man! (Expresses astonishment.)
For heaven's sake! (That can't be true.)
Sigh! Sigh! (Taken from the speech bubbles of comic strips.)
Also in the language of young people: cool, awesome, great.
Source: L. Fouad: *The interjections in German and Arabic from functional-pragmatic view*, Cairo, 2019, pp.270-271.

The following illustration summarises everything we have said about primary and secondary interjections. It should also contribute to a better understanding.

Figure 5: *Classification of primary and secondary interjections*

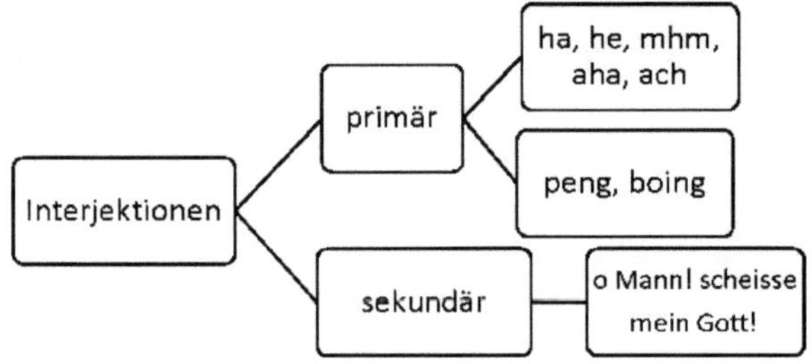

Source: Illustrated by me I.B. Koffi.

This section has allowed us to get an overview of the primary and secondary interjections in German. In the following section, the functions of some German interjections are presented.

1.1.3.3 Function of German interjections

In this section, we will show the functions of German interjections according to their category. Due to their large number, we will limit ourselves to a few symptom interjections (sentiment words) that are used most frequently.

These are explained in detail in this order: *Ah, wow, au, ei, hm, uh, ih, igitt, hurra, juhu, nanu, tja, oje, uff, ach.* All these descriptions have been collected in the digital dictionary of the German language[20] .

The interjection *"ah"* goes well with the expression of joy, astonishment, surprise, sudden understanding, speechlessness and the expression of sighing. It expresses a positive surprise in a falling tone, e.g. *welcome, ah! you are this Anna from the ivory coast.* It can also be used to express satisfaction; for example, after you have eaten a good meal and are finally full, you can say *"ah"*. *"Ah"* in the rising-falling tone refers to a surprise, in this case to something you weren't expecting. This also applies to the interjection *"oh "*.

As far as surprise is concerned, there are many other interjections in the German

[20] Meaning of the German interjection, online at https://www.dwds.de/, last accessed on 24/04/2023, at 13:16.

language. In addition to the interjections already mentioned *(ah, oh)*, Germans also use the interjection *"wow"* to show astonishment in the face of a fact. It's like saying: *"I'm speechless"* or even *"I'm lost for words!"* Let's take an example:
- *Do you know? This man trained for five years to be able to run so fast.*
-*Wow!*
The interjection *"au"* expresses the speaker's physical sensation of pain. It is normally spoken with a falling tone. There are also other variants such as *"aua"* or *"auweia "*, e.g. *au, that hurts*! It is also used to express sudden astonishment or fright.
The interjection *"ei"* expresses surprise and concern. In a dialogue, for example, it can be used to comfort a person who is in pain, and this often happens with children. If a child expresses their pain with *"au"*, parents can comfort them with *"ei"*, which is often accompanied by gestures.
"Hm" expresses a thought process, it can also be equated with the idea of agreement, satisfaction or even doubt. It is difficult to immediately recognise the meaning of this interjection as it sometimes leads to confusion. However, depending on the tone of voice in which it is used, the expressed idea can be recognised. In rising-falling tone refers to a positive flavour. The rising tone corresponds to a doubt or astonishment and in the level tone, reflection of the speaker.
The interjection *"uh "* is sometimes used for coldness in a falling tone. For example: *uuuh, how cold it is!* The interjection *"uh"* also has a negative meaning (repulsion, disgust, horror). It occurs when you are frightened, in a short and sharply falling tone. The interjection *"huch"* with a falling tone also goes with fright.
The interjections *"ih"* and *"igitt"* are used to express disgust. With *"ih"* you have a rising and falling tone. The interjection *"igitt"* intensifies the feeling of disgust. It really shows that you are disgusted and is used with a falling tone. The interjections *"pfui"* and *"brr"* also go with the same feelings.
The interjections *"hurray"* and *"yay"* are purely positive interjections. They radiate feelings of joy, enthusiasm and jubilation. They are expressed with an amplified sound. They are usually used in a festive or joyful context and are usually accompanied by gestures. For example, people are in a stadium to watch their football team play. When the team wins, they can exclaim: *hurraaa! yay*! These interjections are usually prolonged with a similar tone of voice.
"Nanu" can express astonishment, doubt, approval, surprise or even amazement through the tonal accompaniment, the drawl. However, it appears less frequently in everyday speech and generally with a falling-rising tone pattern. Colloquially, the interjection *"nanu"* is used in the double form *"na, na"*.
The interjection *"Well"* denotes thoughtfulness, misgivings, embarrassment or resignation. It is often used in conversation to suggest a sceptical pause for thought. Even when something bad happens and you accept the outcome. *"Well"* is also used to express schadenfreude.
A corruption of the Latin *"o Jesus"*, the German interjection *"oje"* expresses a negative surprise (shock, dismay, pity), e.g. *oje! ich habe mir die Hand verletzt!*

The interjection *"uff"* is mostly used to show physical or mental effort. It also works well to express relief, e.g. *uff ! we have finally arrived.* To express the same feeling, the interjection *"puh"* is used.
The interjection *"ach"*, like many of the interjections already mentioned, expresses different feelings, such as astonishment, suffering, attention, interest, disinterest, bewilderment. Expressions such as *"ach so", "ach ja?", "ach was"* are very common.
The above explanations emphasise that every emotion (sensation) is accompanied by certain interjections. The interjections presented here are only a small part of the interjections that occur in German. Some interjections have foreign origins, but most are purely German. Their use is therefore governed by the rules of belonging to the Germanic sphere. For people who do not belong to it and therefore habitually use interjections from another language, it would be difficult to use those of the German language correctly. This can even lead to interference, as in the case of German students at the University of Felix Houpho^t-Boigny, who usually use other interjections in their languages instead of those of the German language.
To learn more about this, the term interference is summarised below.

1.2 On the term "interference"

With the diversity of languages and the globalisation of the world, contact between people with different languages is becoming increasingly visible. However, the influence of individual languages sometimes leads to interference in linguistic contact. But what is meant by "interference"?
The word "interference" is a derived foreign word and comes from the Latin words *inter* (between) and *ferire* (to strike) and means to overlap, to influence each other.
In linguistics, the term interference refers *to the influence of one linguistic system on another (for example when learning a foreign language)*[21] . Linguistic interference occurs when the influence of one language is visible in the speech of a second language. This is the case, for example, when there is often an unconscious adaptation of a sound to the phonetic system of one language when speaking another language, or when a certain term from the source language penetrates the target language.
Here, too, reference should be made to Josiane Hamers and Michel Blanc, who comment on this as follows: *"Des problemes d'apprentissage dans lesquels l'apprenant transfere le plus souvent inconsciemment et de faqon inappropriee des ëlëments et des traits d'une langue connu a une langue cible."*[22] Linguistic interference generally occurs when two or more languages are used side by side. In contrast to borrowing, which refers to a process of complete or partial adoption of the linguistic features of another language by users of a particular language, interference is an unintentional act. Borrowing can represent linguistic enrichment, i.e. it enables a

[21] Definition of "interference", online at Hhttps://en.thefreedictionary.com/Interference Accessed on 20/03/2023 at 10:55.
[22] H. Josiane / Blanc. M cited by Assia Laidoudi: *Origine des interferences interlinguales lexicales dans les productions ecrites des apprenants de FLE*, Universitat M'SILA, 2020, p.29 : *"Learning problems in which the learner usually unconsciously and inappropriately transfers elements and features of a known language to a target language"*. Translated by me, I.B Koffi.

language to maintain its vitality, renew itself and develop further, whereas interference is seen as a linguistic error. The two terms should therefore not be confused.

The term "interference" is still used as a synonym for "negative transfer". So if you use terms or formulae from language A in language B without this being an error, you are dealing with a positive transfer. For example, the sentence *"I have 12"* instead of *"I am 12"* to say age is a negative transfer from French to German.

Josiane Hamer's[23] also mentions two main causes of language interference, namely limited knowledge of the foreign language. The fact that we do not fully master a language or come into contact with a language for the first time can lead to us introducing terms from our mother tongue into this language. The author also presents psychotypology. According to Hamers, the partial similarity of terms from a previously acquired language with those of a newly learnt language leads users to interfere with them unconsciously.

The words interlingual and intralingual interference, which are explained in the following sections, are subcategorisations of the term.

1.2.1 What is interlingual interference?

Also known as internal interference or interstructural interference, "interlingual interference" refers to the influence of native language components on a foreign language. In interlingual interference, two or more different languages must therefore be taken into account. This means that elements from a language A are used in a language B or words from a language A are used in a language C. Interlingual errors can occur in different areas of the language. For example, there are phonological errors, lexico-semantic errors, morphological errors, syntactic errors and content errors. Phonological errors refer to the poor pronunciation of a word in a given language. Let's take the German word *"Vater"* as an example. Normally, the letter *"v"* in German is pronounced [fau]. However, a young French speaker will read [va:tu] instead of ['fa:tu] because the pronunciation of this letter differs from the pronunciation in his native language.

Lexico-semantic errors refer to the use of an incorrect lexeme (word) or an incorrect word meaning in the language context. A lexico-semantic error occurs, for example, when someone *says "I do sport"* instead of *"I do sport"*. Morphological errors affect the formation of words. Syntactic errors can be described as word order errors, while content errors are pronunciations whose content is incorrect. Interlingual interference is clearly different from intralingual interference. This difference will be demonstrated below.

1.2.2 What is intralingual interference?

While interlingual interference refers to the transfer of the language system of a native language or a learnt language into another language, intralingual interference refers to errors within the same language. According to Karin Kleppin, intralingual errors or intrastructural errors result from three processes, namely overgeneralisation,

[23] Ibid, p. 32.

regularisation and simplification[24] . Overgeneralisation refers to the extension of a rule to phenomena that do not apply to it, for example: *playing music instead of making music*. Regularisation refers to the irregular phenomena of a language that a learner habitually uses, e.g. the use of regular and irregular verbs, whereby all verbs are usually conjugated in the simple regular form, for example*: Bekommen- hat bekommt (instead of hat hat bekommen*). Simplification differs from the other processes in that a complex structure of the target language is avoided. As with interlingual interference, intralingual errors therefore occur in orthography, morphology and syntax.

It is clear that interference is a recurring phenomenon in language use. Having tackled the concepts of "interjection" and "interference", we will now analyse Grice's theory, which will be helpful for the treatment of the practical part of the work.

1.3 . Overview of Grice's theory

The English philosopher Paul Grice is one of the linguists who have focussed their research on discourse. In 1968, Grice conceived the so-called "co-operation principle"[25] , in which the author mentioned the prerequisites for successful communication. In it, Grice elaborated four maxims, the main idea of which can be summarised in the following questions: What is important in communication between dialogue partners? What should be taken into account? Or what plays an important role in communication?

The maxims elaborated by Grice are, in a sense, rules that dialogue partners must adhere to in their conversation in order to communicate successfully. Firstly, Grice mentions the maxim of quantity, which aims to get straight to the point in a conversation (as necessary and not talking too much), secondly the maxim of quality, which is about getting the right thing out. The maxim of relation, which emphasises relevance, is also part of this. Finally comes the maxim of modality, which refers to clarity.

In addition, Grice emphasises important factors that are taken into account in the conversation between speech partners (speaker and listener). These include the context of action and the place of action. For Grice, grammatical rules are not really essential for the successful realisation of a communication. The intention that the author pursues with his statements is the most important thing. We present the principle of co-operation more clearly as follows:

Paul Grice defines language as a functional system that is orientated towards a specific intention. Language is therefore a means of expression that aims to realise a speaker's intention and at the same time has an effect on the other person. In order to make oneself understood and achieve the goal of the speech act, certain norms must be adhered to. Paul Grice therefore speaks of the co-operation principle. This is understood to mean that the speaker's utterances must be consistent with what is expected of him when he intervenes in a discourse whose goal or direction is shared by

[24] K. Karin quoted by Nguyen Thi OANH: *Intralingual interference on the morphosyntactic errors of Vietnamese German students at level B1*, University of Hanoi, 2018, p. 237.

[25] Cooperation principle, online at https://www.grin.com/document/338660, last accessed on 22 May. 2023, at 7: 39.

the interlocutors. In other words, recognising the speaker's intention is therefore a necessary and sufficient condition for successful communication.

This theory is well suited to explain the inappropriate use of interjections in the speech of German students at the University of Felix Houpho^t-Boigny.

PART II

PRACTICAL PART OF THE WORK

2. analysis of incorrect use of German interjections in the speech of 1st year German students (2021-2022) at the University of Felix H()iiph()iii t-Boigny

The analysis below highlights the interjections used by first-year German students at the University of Felix I Iouplioiic t-Boigny. It was noted that they do not take into account the interjections of the learning language (German) in their conversation.

In order to understand the linguistic features underlying the incorrect use of interjections, a questionnaire was distributed to around 50 students. In the questionnaire, the students were given an exercise in which they were asked to respond to various statements with the appropriate interjections. In order to be able to better interpret the results, only the reactions of 24 of the students surveyed are taken into account in our analysis. Based on this questionnaire, the analysis is elaborated as follows:

First and foremost, the interjections expressing sympathy are analysed. Secondly, we analyse the interjections expressing astonishment and finally we focus on the interjections expressing joy.

2.1 Interjection to express empathy: case study of the interjections "*Yako*" and "*eh*"

Here attention is drawn to the interjections used by the students on the questionnaire to express empathy. The responses shown are only 12 of those obtained during our research with 50 first year students. Among the interjections used, two different interjections appeared several times. These are the interjections *"yako"* and *"eh"*. These are therefore analysed one after the other.

2.1.1 Case study of the interjection *"yako"*

In the first step of this analysis, we will look at the use of the interjection *"yako"* by 1st year German students. For this purpose, the reactions of eight students were taken into consideration.

Statement: My mum died yesterday. My sister wrote to me.

Reactions from students:

Student 1: *hum! Yako*

Student 2: *how!!! Yako*

Student 3: *truly yako all my sincere condolences.*

Student 4: *haa yako!*

Student 5: *yako*

Student 6: *oh oh yako*

Student 7: *yako, I am sad.*

Student 8: *oh my god! yako*

The example above shows different reactions of students to a sad statement. It can be seen here that the majority of students reacted with *"yako"*. These students have thereby expressed empathy. In some statements, the word *"yako"* was accompanied by additional interjections such as *"hum"*, *"haa", "oh", "ha", "how"*. But what is meant by *"yako"*?

The word *"yako "* comes from the Baoule language[26] and is an interjection, so to speak. Although it has its origins in the Baoule language, the interjection *"yako"* is used by foreign Ivorians. This allows them to express their support or sympathy for an unfortunate situation to the person they are talking to.

This makes it clear that the interjection *"yako"* is not tied to the German language. In other words, the interjection learnt by the German students does not fit German. As a rule, the students were supposed to react as follows: *"oh!", "oh no!" "I'm sorry"* or even *"oh dear", "my condolences"*. In contrast, most students did not pay attention to the correct interjections. However, this mode of expression can be explained pragmalinguistically.

In fact, pragmatics states that a statement can be understood contextually. This means that the understanding of a statement is not necessarily based on the rules, but on the context of communication. Those students who respond with *"yako"* certainly pay attention to the circumstances of the shared utterance. The aim of expressing the interjection *"yako"* is to communicate a good intention to the language recipient. In this way, students want to show that they sympathise with the message they are being told. Although the interpreted interjection does not originate from German, it fits the situation well.

Also following Grice with the co-operation principle, it is obvious that the students concerned take sociolinguistic factors into account when using the interjection *"yako"*, namely the place of action. Since the students concerned share a common culture with their interlocutor, they are appropriate to use the interjection *"yako"* conventionally, otherwise the message with German interjections would certainly have carried a different weight and would have led to misunderstanding. Thus, although some students used German terms such as *"oh my God"* and *"really"*, they still used the interjection *"yako"* to emphasise their distress. This can be clearly seen in the third and eighth students. With the interjection *"yako"*, the language recipient can thus understand the intention of the language producer and in turn react well according to this intention.

Below is an illustration that helps us to see clearly the different aspects that are taken into account in a conversation and even influence the way German students express themselves.

[26] Cote d'Ivoire has over 60 local languages and the Baoule language is one of them.

of German students. This is especially true for the interjections to be analysed next.

Figure 6: *Matrix of the interaction process between language producers and language recipients*

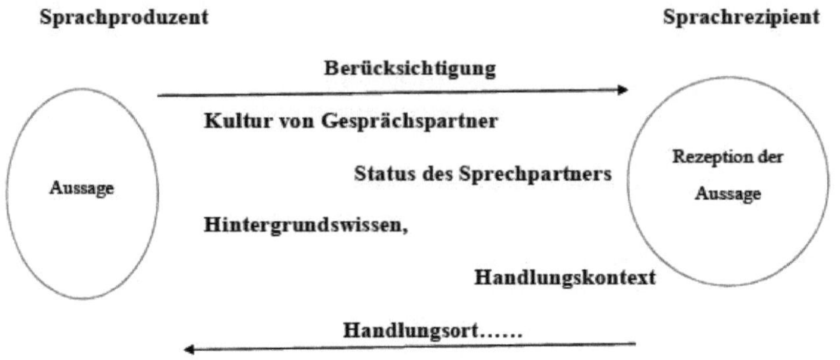

Language producer Language recipient
Consideration
Culture of dialogue partners Reception of the

Status of the interlocutor
Statement
Background knowledge,
Context of action
Place of action

Source: Illustrated by me I. B. Koffi.

The diagram shows various parameters that are taken into account when two or more people communicate. To be more precise, the speakers speak on the basis of their culture and background knowledge. The context of action, the place of action and the status of speaking partners are also of great importance. This explains why German students tend to use Ivorian interjections instead of German interjections. Instead of saying *"oh no", "oje"*, they *use "yako"*, which is typical for Ivorians and fits the empathy towards the interlocutor. Since the interlocutor was identified as Ivorian in the questionnaire, they referred to a colloquial interjection to show their feeling.

In order to distribute their empathy, the students used other interjections in the questionnaire, which is subject to analysis.

2.1.2 Case study of the interjection *"eh"*

In our questionnaire, the interjection *"eh"* was used in passing. This is what this analysis refers to.

Statement: My mum died yesterday. My sister wrote to me.

Reactions from students:

Student 1: *eeeh yako*

Student 2: *eh!*

Student 3: *eeeh! Too bad!*

Student 4*: euhh*

The interjection *yako* was generally used by the majority in the questionnaire, but the interjection *"eh"* was also used. This interjection is particularly requested here. Instead of simply writing *"eh"*, some students used a variant "*eeeh*". Like *"yako"*, this interjection does not originate from German. The interjection *"eh"* is rather used in some Ivorian local languages and expresses contextually different feelings: astonishment, pain, sympathy, disenchantment, discouragement, regret and sometimes serves to warn or address someone about something. The intonation of this interjection sometimes takes into account the context in which it is used. Most of the time, the interjection *"eh"* is elongated in its use and sometimes strongly emphasised.

The interjection "*eh* " also occurs in the French language, which is incidentally the official language of the country. Another spelling is "*κë"*. In French, it also refers to admiration, surprise or even pain. We can visualise this as follows:

Figure 7: *Use of the interjection "eh" in French and in local languages of Cdte d'Ivoire*

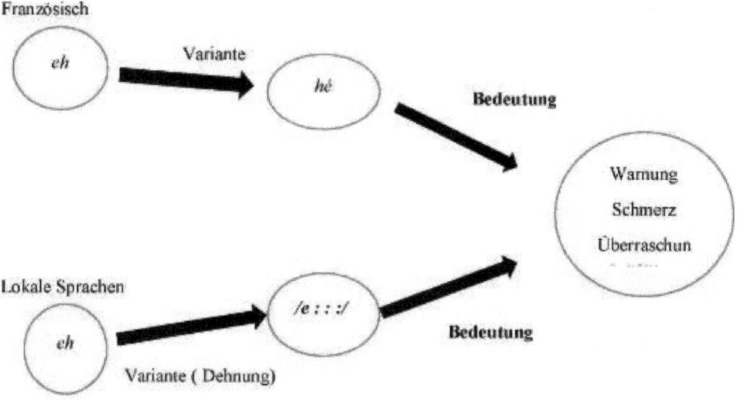

Quelle: Von mir I. B. Koffi abgebildet.

Thanks to this illustration, we understand how the interjection *"eh"* is common among Ivorians. It appears not only in local languages, but also in French, the official language of the country. Here too, as in the first case study, we are dealing with incorrect usage, because the German interjection that had to be used in such a context is not this one. This is due to the fact that the students are reacting to habit. The influence of the French language and the local languages had an effect on the language of communication (German).

The interviewees live in Cote d'Ivoire and are used to expressing themselves in this way in sad situations. This fact has such a great influence on the language of learning that they even use routine interjections in this language. The culture is emphasised here in an unconscious way.

Figure 8: *Effect of Ivorian interjections on German*

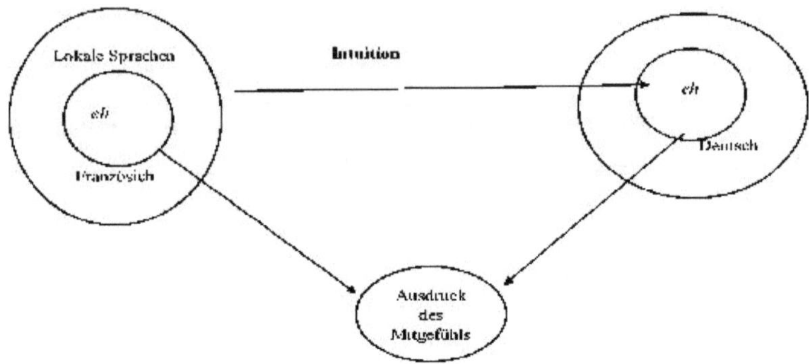

Source: Illustrated by I.B. Koffi.

The illustration above supports what we have explained. We can see here how the same interjection GefuhlsmaBig occurs in different languages.

The use of the interjections *"yako"* and *"eh"* reveals a sense of empathy. It is noted that the German interjections are not taken into account by the students. In order to express empathy, they paid attention to interjections in their own languages. What about interjections to express astonishment? This is the subject of the following section.

2.2 Interjection to express astonishment

In our questionnaires with the first-year students, they were confronted with a situation during the exercise in which they were asked to express themselves with astonishment. In other words, they were asked to express astonishment. The results obtained are then the subject of the following analysis. A total of 5 reactions were observed here.

Statement: do you know? I read in the newspaper yesterday that homosexuality could soon be legalised in the Ivory Coast. Yes, I'm a bit surprised, but I still think it's great!

Reactions from students:

Student 1*: Hum! Cannot do well*

Student 2*: Hein!!! That's not good*

Student 3*: hum? Unfortunately I think differently*

Student 4*: are you crazy?*

Student 5*: o are you mad?*

When expressing astonishment, it was found that the 1st year German studies students hardly use any German interjections. Of the 50 students surveyed, only 10 were able to use German interjections such as *"ach so"?, "wirklich?", "Sicher?"* . Since they could not use the appropriate interjections, about 30 students resorted to making sentences and throwing swear words to show their dissatisfaction.

Most of the students assessed therefore opted for foreign interjections, namely *"hum"* and *"hein".* In the Ivorian language, these interjections refer to astonishment, deliberation, reflection or doubt. The meaning depends above all on the situation and the intonation of the interjection. In French and even in German, the interjection *"hum"* in particular can be equated with the interjection *"hm"*, which also expresses the same feelings, namely reflection, doubt or even astonishment. However, the interjection *"hein"* is not found at all in the German language and cannot be equated with any interjection. As homosexuality is almost a taboo subject in Côte d'Ivoire, it can be concluded that the people concerned reacted in this way to show their astonishment. However, the students of German studies are talking in German, so the intoned reactions (*hem!!!, hum? Hum!)* are incorrect. They are not appropriate to the German language. These interjections are more in keeping with the Ivorian language. It would have been conceivable to use interjections such as "*really*?" *"Really*?" or "*oje" instead.* So how can this usage be explained?

If you analyse the circumstances and the students' reactions, you can see that they are still influenced by their linguistic environment. The spelling of the interjections used is also proof of this:

Hum = used in the Ivorian language ***hm*** = used in German

Source: Illustrated by me I.B. Koffi.

Following Paul Grice's maxims that the participants in a conversation should speak in order to be understood (relevance, clarity), it is obvious that the use of German interjections had led the interlocutor to think rather than to understand. The use of Ivorian interjections (*hein, hum*), which are well known to the interlocutors, therefore makes it easier to convey the message. As Grice's theory has shown, the speaker's intention overrides the linguistic theory. Much more important is the effect that his statement could have on the other person. If the student responded with *"really?", or "really?"*, he had not been able to communicate to his counterpart that he was very surprised. He would have been less interested in the conversation insofar as they both (language producer and language recipient) have their own language code.

The special nature of languages can also be mentioned. Since languages are cultural tools, the way in which people express themselves differs. Interjections are also part of the language and differ from one language to another.

language to another, they are, so to speak, linked to habit. So students are influenced by this cultural habit. Everything that has been said can be schematised as follows:

Figure 9: *Consideration of culture when using interjections in the conversation of German students.*

Interjections from normal conversation

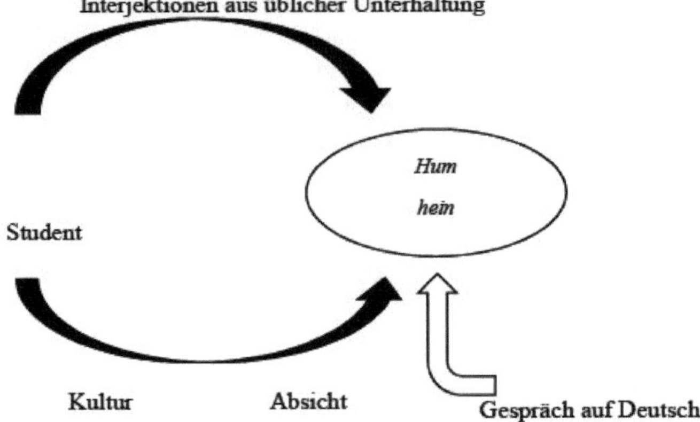

Student *Hum hein*

Culture Intention Speech in German

Source: Illustrated by I.B. Koffi.

As already mentioned, first-year German students find it difficult to use typical German interjections to express their astonishment. This time, the following analysis focuses on the expression of joy.

2.3 Interjection to express joy

In addition to empathy and amazement, first year students were also asked to express satisfaction with what they were told in the same exercise. The results are analysed in this section. After we have presented them, their use will be justified.

Statement: Hello, you've passed all your exams, and so have I!

Reactions from students:

Student 1: *yes ahn! That's great*

Student 2: *waouu!*

Student 3: *brilliant!*

Student 4: *hum! I do not believe*

Student 5: *it's great*

Student 6: *God has shown mercy, thank you brother.*

Student 7: *I am very satisfied, I was a bit surprised because it was difficult*

The students find themselves in a situation where they have been given some good news. They have been told that they have successfully passed their exams at the university. It should be noted that different interjections were used by the students to communicate their happiness. The reactions of 7 students were taken into account for

the analysis.
In the first selected reaction, the use of the interjection *"ahn"* is recorded. The second contains another interjection: *"waouu"*. The third and fourth interjections are: *"gonial"*, *"hum!"*. The others did not use any interjections. It should also be noted that in the first and fourth students, the learnt interjections *"ahn "* and *"hm "* are accompanied by sentences. The second and third students only threw interjections without adding sentences, so they all express a positive feeling or joy. As I said, they are happy about the good results in the exam. The last one, however, forms a sentence with German words.
However, all the interjections used by the students are not from German. The interjection *"ahn"* is used by the Ivorians and expresses either surprise or joy, depending on the context and tone pattern. It can also be written *"han"*. Here in particular, the language producer is certainly surprised by the result, but he is pleased and the following sentence *"that's great"* shows it quite clearly. In thc second case, the student also prints a kind of surprise, but as with the first student, this refers to joy, this interjection is required, otherwise one would have simply written *"waou"*. The printed interjection comes from French.
The "ðëmal" printed by the student can also be found in the French language. if it was written *"genial"*, it could have matched the German. But here the spelling is typically French. As with the first reaction, the student has unfortunately not taken the German interjection into account. In the last response selected for analysis, a typical Ivorian interjection can be noted. We can therefore see from these results that the students used Ivorian and French interjections. None of them used the appropriate interjection.
These German interjections to express joy are called *oh! hurra, juhu! Super! Spitze*! These interjections should normally be used by the students, they are quite positive and fit well with the expression of joy. But how can this be explained? Why weren't the German interjections taken into account here?
These are spontaneous reactions. The student is not aware that he is talking in German and should therefore use a German interjection. He reacts with the first intention that comes to him, namely to show his satisfaction. The use of the interjection is therefore not fixed to a learnt rule. Here too, the first language of the person concerned influences the use of interjections. In addition, Paul Grice is of the opinion that the language recipient must take the co-operation principle into account in the interaction. It assumes that the language producer expects an action from the language recipient. This therefore requires some statements that take into account the culture and prior knowledge of the protagonists. Because the students have a common language code, they would not have understood each other if a different interjection had been used, even if it expressed joy. As with the expression of sympathy and astonishment, the students' first language also has a major influence on joy. They may speak a different language, but they still refer to their first language to communicate their feelings.
In this paper, we have analysed the interjections used by first-year students (2021-2022) to express emotions such as compassion, astonishment and joy. What conclusions can we draw from this analysis?

Balance of the analysis

The practical part of our research focused on analysing the incorrect use of interjections in the speech of German students at the University of Felix Houpho^t-Boigny. This results in the following:

It was observed in the analysis that most of the interjections used by the first-year German students have an Ivorian origin. These form the majority of the interjections used in the questionnaire. When one speaks of Ivorian origin, one refers both to the Ivorian colloquial language and to the local languages.

For the most part, the interjections *"yako" and "eh"* were used in the questionnaires to express sympathy. Only some students chose to use fir German interjections, including: *"oh my God".* The interjections *"hein"* and *"hum"* were mostly used to express astonishment and the interjections *"waou", "hum"* and *"genial"* were used to express joy. The German interjections considered here form only a small part of the interjections used. Especially when expressing astonishment and joy, they use sentences instead of interjections to express their feelings.

The repeated use of interjections that are foreign to German shows that the German students are influenced by their mother tongues and their culture. It can also be attributed to the fact that the students concerned try to be understood by their interlocutor.

Conclusion

Our research, entitled: Incorrect use of interjections in the speech of first-year German students (20212022) at the University of Felix Houpho^t-Boigny, was mainly concerned with identifying linguistic features underlying the inappropriate use of interjections by some German students. This gave rise to the following central question:

What are the psycholinguistic characteristics related to the incorrect use of interjections in 1st year German students at the University of Fëlix Houpho^t-Boigny?

After the analysis, it can therefore be confirmed that the German students concerned are influenced in their conversations by their mother tongues and their culture. The need to be understood by the interlocutor is also a reason for the incorrect use of interjections in their conversations. As they are used to using interjections that are specific to their culture and environment, it is difficult for 1st year German students to refer to interjections in the language they are studying (German).

Thanks to this research, we have been able to address an obvious phenomenon that has long left many people indifferent. This research has led to German students, especially first year students, developing a great interest in German interjections. Although these are culturally conditioned, we believe it is important that German students pay more attention to the interjections of the language of learning and use them in their conversations. The present research is seen as a stimulus for further research, including punctuation errors among German students in Côte d'Ivoire.

BIBLIOGRAPHY

1. Primary literature

The questionnaires I conducted with the 1st year German students (2021-2022) at the University of Felix Houpho^t-Boigny.

2. Secondary literature

AGNIMEL, S. Augustin : *L'enseignement de I'allemand dans les lycëes et colleges de Cdte d'Ivoire : Etude critique des mëthodes utilisëes pour I'enseignement de la langue et des contenus proposes en civilisation dans les manuels (1958-1992).* Doctoral thesis, supervised by Prof Jean Moes, Metz, 1994.

ASSIA, Laidoudi : *Origine des interjections interlinguales lexicales dans les productions ëcrites des apprenants de FLE,* Universitat MSILA, 2020.

BADI, H. Saddam : *le franqais parE au mali : interfërence du bambara dans le franqais (une ëtude linguistique et comparative)*, Universitat AL-Mustansiriya, 2020.

CARON-PARGUE, Josiane/ CARON Jean : *Les interjections comme marqueurs du fonctionnement cognitif,* in "cahiers de praxematique", Universitat Poitiers, 2000.

CLIFF, Goddard: *Interjections and emotions (with special reference to "suprise" and "disgust")*, Queensland, 2014.

EHLICH, Konrad*: Interjections.* Tubingen : Max Niemeyer Verlag, 1986.

FERAR, Driss : *L'influence de la culture sur la pratique des MRH. Qualitative study.* Quartage: EMS Verlag, 2017.

FOUAD, Lobna*: The interjections in German and Arabic from a functional-pragmatic point of view*, Cairo, 2019.

NORDGREN, Lars : *Greek Interjections : syntax, semantics and pragmatics*. Berlin: De Gruyter Verlag, 2015.

GUTZMANN, Daniel: *Linguistik der Expressivitat,* University of Cologne: Institute for German Language and Literature I, 2015.

HORVAT, Ana: *Use of phrasemes and interjections in German and Croatian youth magazines*. Master's thesis, supervised by Dr sc. Anita Pavic Pintaric, University of Zadar, 2018.

HUESMAN, Ilka: *Punctuation and intonation of interjections in German*. Mercator Institute for Language Learning and German as a Second Language, University of Cologne, 2021.

KCHAOU, M. Ksouri : *les Interfërences linguistiques dans le langage communautaire des banlieues tunisiennes*, Universitat Carthage, 2013-2014.

KOSCH, Nathalie: "*Interjections and onomatopoeias in Polish": An investigation of everyday use in the age of electronic communication*, Vienna, 2015.

OANH, Nguyen Thi: *Intralingual interference on the morphosyntactic errors of Vietnamese German students at level B1*, University of Hanoi, 2018.

PROSKE, Nadine: *On the function and classification of language-organising imperatives*. In "Discourse markers in German". Gottingen: Verlag fur Gesprachsforschung, 2017.

REBER, Elisabeth/ COUPER-KUHLEN, Elizabeth: *Interjections between lexicon and vocalisation: lexeme or sound object?* Berlin: De Gruyter Verlag, 2010.

STOLE, Hildegunn: *Interjections in Late Middle English play texts: A multi-variable approach.* PhD thesis, supervised by Prof. Merja Stenroos, University of Stavanger, 2012.

YANG, Chaiqin: *Interjections and onomatopoeias in language comparison: German versus Chinese.* Doctoral thesis, supervised by Prof. Dr Ulrich Rebstock, Freiburg, 2001.

3. Other literature

DUDEN: *German Universal Dictionary A-Z.* Duden Verlag, Mannheim, 1996.

DUDEN: *Etymological dictionary of German words*. Berlin: Akademie Verlag GmbH, 1993.

LUBKE, Diethard: *Schulgrammatik Deutsch: Vom Beispiel zur Regel*, Berlin: Corneseln Verlag, 1999.

4. Internet sources

Number of German learners in Africa, online at https://amp-dw.com:de:afrika-deutsch-als-trendsprache/a-54465700, last accessed on 30 January 2023, at 12:25.

BALDAUF-QUILIATRE, Heike: *Worter, die keine sind*, Lyon, 2013, online at HALId: halshs-00830272https://shs.hal.science/halshs-00830272, last accessed on 10. 04.2023, at 15: 16.

Meaning of the German interjection, online at hhtps://www.dwds.de/, last accessed on 24/04/2023, at 13:16.

CHUKWUDI, Awa: *Interfërence linguistique chez les ëtudiants universitaires de la deuxieme anni'e de Nnamdiaziweuniversity :cas de l'emploi du verbe " etre "*,Nnamdiaziweuniversity Awka, 2002, online at http://www.jmelnau.com.ng, last accessed on 12/07/2023, at 1: 25.

Definition of interference, online at Hhtps://en.thefreedictionary. com/Interference, last accessed on 20/03/2023, at 10:55.

FAUST, Johann: *Functional analysis of the lexeme "krass" as an interjection of youth language, Munich.* GRIN Verlag, 2020, online at https://www.grin.com/document/,letzter Accessed on 02/07/2023 at 21:00.

FRAISSE, Amel / PAROUBEK, Patrick: *Les interjections pour dëtecter les emotions,* Caen, 2015, online at https:/hal.science/hal-0161718-, last accessed on 29/03/2023, at 21:04.

HALTE, Pierre : *Positionnement syntaxique des interjections et des emoticdnes : modalisation, portee, visee.* In "cahiers de praxematiques", 2018, online at https//shs.hal.science/halshs-01803669, last accessed on 11/07/2023, at 23:13.

Interjection types, online at wortwuchs.net/gramm atik/interjektion, last accessed on 20/08/2020, at 9:19.

Cooperation principle, online at https://www.grin.com/document/338660, last accessed on 22 May. 2023, at 7: 39.

MELLI, Angelo: *The co-operation principle of Herbert Paul Grice. Analysis of advertising language with regard to the maxim of conversation,* online at

https:/:www.grin.com/document/338660, last accessed on 22 May 2023, at 15:30.
MEILER, Matthias/ HUYNH, Ilham: *The interjection boah in everyday payments. Eine Annaherung anhand von face-to-face und Instant-Messaging-Kommunikation*, 2020, online at hhtps://dx.doi.org/10.13092/lo.104.7289, last accessed on 12 July 2023, at 1: 52.
WIEMER, O. Rudolf : *Beispiele zur deutschen Grammatik,* Wolfgang Fietkau Verlag, Berlin 1971,online at http s ://www. stichter.c om/ show/interkulturell es-lernen/episode:interkulturelles-lernen-gedicht-empfindungsworter-von-rudolf-otto-wiemer-62035764, last accessed on 29 March 2023, at 22:02.

ANNEX

Situation A : Du sprichst mit deinem Freund, der nun in Deutschland lebt. Er kündigt dir seine Ankunft nach Heimat an. Wie reagierst du ?

X : Hallo ! Wie geht es dir ?

Du : Danke! Und du?

X : Mir geht es leider nicht gut.

Du :.. Was passiert

X : Meine Mutter ist gestern gestorben. Meine Schwester hat mir geschrieben.

Du :.. Rau!!! Yaka

X : Ich komme also bald zu Hause.

Du :..o.k

X : Vielen Dank .

Situation B : Einer deiner Freunde der Deutsch-Abteilung ruft dich an und erzählt dir eine Nachricht. Wie reagierst du

Freund Y

Y : Hallo mein(e) Freund(in),alles gut ?

Du :..Hallo! ya und du?

Y : Weißt du ? Ich habe gestern in der Zeitung gelesen, dass Homosexualität in der Elfenbeinküste bald legalisiert werden könnte.

Du :..Nein! er ist falsch

Y : Ja, ich bin ein bisschen überrascht, aber ich finde es trotzdem toll !

Du :..oh mein gott

Situation C : Dein bester Freund ruft dich an und informiert dich über die Ergebnisse der akademischen Prüfungen. Wie reagierst du darauf ?

Freund Z

Z : Hallo ! Du hast alle Prüfungen bestanden, ich auch.

Du :..gott..sei Dank!

Situation A : Du sprichst mit deinem Freund, der nun in Deutschland lebt. Er kündigt dir seine Ankunft nach Heimat an. Wie reagierst du ?

X : Hallo ! Wie geht es dir ?

Du : Es geht's mir gut

X : Mir geht es leider nicht gut.

Du : Warum ,

X : Meine Mutter ist gestern gestorben. Meine Schwester hat mir geschrieben.

Du : Eintschuldigung

X : Ich komme also bald zu Hause.

Du : Ich warte dir

X : Vielen Dank .

Situation B : Einer deiner Freunde der Deutsch-Abteilung ruft dich an und erzählt dir eine Nachricht. Wie reagierst du

Freund Y

Y : Hallo mein(e) Freund(in),alles gut ?

Du : Ya

Y : Weißt du ? Ich habe gestern in der Zeitung gelesen, dass Homosexualität in der Elfenbeinküste bald legalisiert werden könnte.

Du : Das ist nicht Richtig !

Y : Ja, ich bin ein bisschen überrascht, aber ich finde es trotzdem toll !

Du : O Bist du Verrük Wahnsinn ?

Situation C : Dein bester Freund ruft dich an und informiert dich über die Ergebnisse der akademischen Prüfungen. Wie reagierst du darauf ?

Freund Z

Z : Hallo ! Du hast alle Prüfungen bestanden, ich auch.

Du : Haa, ich bin zufrieden, aber habe ich nicht alle bestanden

Situation A : Du sprichst mit deinem Freund, der nun in Deutschland lebt. Er kündigt dir seine Ankunft nach Heimat an. Wie reagierst du ?

X : Hallo ! Wie geht es dir ?

Du : Hallo! mir gut.

X : Mir geht es leider nicht gut.

Du : Warum?

X : Meine Mutter ist gestern gestorben. Meine Schwester hat mir geschrieben.

Du : Hoo! Sorry!

X : Ich komme also bald zu Hause.

Du : ok

X : Vielen Dank .

Situation B : Einer deiner Freunde der Deutsch-Abteilung ruft dich an und erzählt dir eine Nachricht. Wie reagierst du

Freund Y

Y : Hallo mein(e) Freund(in),alles gut ?

Du : Ja!

Y : Weißt du ? Ich habe gestern in der Zeitung gelesen, dass Homosexualität in der Elfenbeinküste bald legalisiert werden könnte.

Du : Vielleicht

Y : Ja, ich bin ein bisschen überrascht, aber ich finde es trotzdem toll !

Du : Ich bin nicht natürlich!

Situation C : Dein bester Freund ruft dich an und informiert dich über die Ergebnisse der akademischen Prüfungen. Wie reagierst du darauf ?

Freund Z

Z : Hallo ! Du hast alle Prüfungen bestanden, ich auch.

Du : ~~Es freut mich~~ génial!

Situation A : Du sprichst mit deinem Freund, der nun in Deutschland lebt. Er kündigt dir seine Ankunft nach Heimat an. Wie reagierst du ?

X : Hallo ! Wie geht es dir ?

Du : gut danke schön und dir

X : Mir geht es leider nicht gut.

Du : Ja

X : Meine Mutter ist gestern gestorben. Meine Schwester hat mir geschrieben.

Du : ah ah Yako

X : Ich komme also bald zu Hause.

Du : ok gott danke.

X : Vielen Dank .

Situation B : Einer deiner Freunde der Deutsch-Abteilung ruft dich an und erzählt dir eine Nachricht. Wie reagierst du

Freund Y

Y : Hallo mein(e) Freund(in),alles gut ?

Du : Ja und du.

Y : Weißt du ? Ich habe gestern in der Zeitung gelesen, dass Homosexualität in der Elfenbeinküste bald legalisiert werden könnte.

Du : das ist nicht correct ich bin nicht zufriede.

Y : Ja, ich bin ein bisschen überrascht, aber ich finde es trotzdem toll !

Du : Nein Wir ich bin nicht zufriede, wenn Homos nicht sehr gut.

Situation C : Dein bester Freund ruft dich an und informiert dich über die Ergebnisse der akademischen Prüfungen. Wie reagierst du darauf ?

Freund Z

Z : Hallo ! Du hast alle Prüfungen bestanden, ich auch.

Du : Aha ok) gott danke.

Situation A : Du sprichst mit deinem Freund, der nun in Deutschland lebt. Er kündigt dir seine Ankunft nach Heimat an. Wie reagierst du ?

X : Hallo ! Wie geht es dir ?

Du : mir geht es gut und du

X : Mir geht es leider nicht gut.

Du : warum ist los ?

X : Meine Mutter ist gestern gestorben. Meine Schwester hat mir geschrieben.

Du : yako, ich bin traurig

X : Ich komme also bald zu Hause.

Du : Ok, ich warte dir

X : Vielen Dank .

Situation B : Einer deiner Freunde der Deutsch-Abteilung ruft dich an und erzählt dir eine Nachricht. Wie reagierst du

Freund Y

Y : Hallo mein(e) Freund(in),alles gut ?

Du : ya, ich bin gut und dir

Y : Weißt du ? Ich habe gestern in der Zeitung gelesen, dass Homosexualität in der Elfenbeinküste bald legalisiert werden könnte.

Du : warum ? ich bin sehr uberrascht

Y : Ja, ich bin ein bisschen überrascht, aber ich finde es trotzdem toll !

Du : Bist du verrückt ?

Situation C : Dein bester Freund ruft dich an und informiert dich über die Ergebnisse der akademischen Prüfungen. Wie reagierst du darauf ?

Freund Z

Z : Hallo ! Du hast alle Prüfungen bestanden, ich auch.

Du : hoch, Super ich bin sehr freu

Situation A : Du sprichst mit deinem Freund, der nun in Deutschland lebt. Er kündigt dir seine Ankunft nach Heimat an. Wie reagierst du ?

X : Hallo ! Wie geht es dir ?

Du : Es geht mir gut und du

X : Mir geht es leider nicht gut.

Du : Warum ?

X : Meine Mutter ist gestern gestorben. Meine Schwester hat mir geschrieben.

Du : Oh mein Gott!, yako

X : Ich komme also bald zu Hause.

Du : Okay

X : Vielen Dank .

Situation B : Einer deiner Freunde der Deutsch-Abteilung ruft dich an und erzählt dir eine Nachricht. Wie reagierst du

Freund Y

Y : Hallo mein(e) Freund(in),alles gut ?

Du : gut und du

Y : Weißt du ? Ich habe gestern in der Zeitung gelesen, dass Homosexualität in der Elfenbeinküste bald legalisiert werden könnte.

Du : Wirklich !

Y : Ja, ich bin ein bisschen überrascht, aber ich finde es trotzdem toll !

Du : bist du verrückt mein Freund

Situation C : Dein bester Freund ruft dich an und informiert dich über die Ergebnisse der akademischen Prüfungen. Wie reagierst du darauf ?

Freund Z

Z : Hallo ! Du hast alle Prüfungen bestanden, ich auch.

Du : Wirklich, Gott Danke

Situation A : Du sprichst mit deinem Freund, der nun in Deutschland lebt. Er kündigt dir seine Ankunft nach Heimat an. Wie reagierst du ?

X : Hallo ! Wie geht es dir ?

Du : Wunderbar! Und dir ?

X : Mir geht es leider nicht gut.

Du : Gut Warum

X : Meine Mutter ist gestern gestorben. Meine Schwester hat mir geschrieben.

Du : Eeeh schade

X : Ich komme also bald zu Hause.

Du : Sei stark

X : Vielen Dank .

Situation B : Einer deiner Freunde der Deutsch-Abteilung ruft dich an und erzählt dir eine Nachricht. Wie reagierst du

Freund Y

Y : Hallo mein(e) Freund(in),alles gut ?

Du : Ja Ja...

Y : Weißt du ? Ich habe gestern in der Zeitung gelesen, dass Homosexualität in der Elfenbeinküste bald legalisiert werden könnte.

Du : Oh... schade

Y : Ja, ich bin ein bisschen überrascht, aber ich finde es trotzdem toll !

Du : Nein !.....

Situation C : Dein bester Freund ruft dich an und informiert dich über die Ergebnisse der akademischen Prüfungen. Wie reagierst du darauf ?

Freund Z

Z : Hallo ! Du hast alle Prüfungen bestanden, ich auch.

Du : Super

Situation A : Du sprichst mit deinem Freund, der nun in Deutschland lebt. Er kündigt dir seine Ankunft nach Heimat an. Wie reagierst du ?

X : Hallo ! Wie geht es dir ?

Du : es geht gute und

X : Mir geht es leider nicht gut.

Du : Hum ! yako !

X : Meine Mutter ist gestern gestorben. Meine Schwester hat mir geschrieben.

Du : bleileid mein Freund

X : Ich komme also bald zu Hause.

Du : Tatsache Aufmerksamkeit

X : Vielen Dank .

Situation B : Einer deiner Freunde der Deutsch-Abteilung ruft dich an und erzählt dir eine Nachricht. Wie reagierst du

Freund Y

Y : Hallo mein(e) Freund(in),alles gut ?

Du : ya alle gute

Y : Weißt du ? Ich habe gestern in der Zeitung gelesen, dass Homosexualität in der Elfenbeinküste bald legalisiert werden könnte.

Du : Hum!....

Y : Ja, ich bin ein bisschen überrascht, aber ich finde es trotzdem toll !

Du : nicht kann gut

Situation C : Dein bester Freund ruft dich an und informiert dich über die Ergebnisse der akademischen Prüfungen. Wie reagierst du darauf ?

Freund Z

Z : Hallo ! Du hast alle Prüfungen bestanden, ich auch.

Du : Hum! Ich nicht glauben

Situation A : Du sprichst mit deinem Freund, der nun in Deutschland lebt. Er kündigt dir seine Ankunft nach Heimat an. Wie reagierst du ?

X : Hallo ! Wie geht es dir ?

Du : Es geht gut

X : Mir geht es leider nicht gut.

Du :. Oh ! Warum

X : Meine Mutter ist gestern gestorben. Meine Schwester hat mir geschrieben.

Du : Eh.. YAKO

X : Ich komme also bald zu Hause.

Du :. OK..

X : Vielen Dank .

Situation B : Einer deiner Freunde der Deutsch-Abteilung ruft dich an und erzählt dir eine Nachricht. Wie reagierst du

Freund Y

Y : Hallo mein(e) Freund(in),alles gut ?

Du :. JA.............

Y : Weißt du ? Ich habe gestern in der Zeitung gelesen, dass Homosexualität in der Elfenbeinküste bald legalisiert werden könnte.

Du :..H.U.M.!.. WARUM

Y : Ja, ich bin ein bisschen überrascht, aber ich finde es trotzdem toll !

Du :. humm

Situation C : Dein bester Freund ruft dich an und informiert dich über die Ergebnisse der akademischen Prüfungen. Wie reagierst du darauf ?

Freund Z

Z : Hallo ! Du hast alle Prüfungen bestanden, ich auch.

Du :. Das.. gefällt mir

Situation A : Du sprichst mit deinem Freund, der nun in Deutschland lebt. Er kündigt dir seine Ankunft nach Heimat an. Wie reagierst du ?

X : Hallo ! Wie geht es dir ?

Du: Gut, und du?

X : Mir geht es leider nicht gut.

Du: Oh! Scheide!

X : Meine Mutter ist gestern gestorben. Meine Schwester hat mir geschrieben.

Du: Euhh!

X : Ich komme also bald zu Hause.

Du: Danke

X : Vielen Dank .

Situation B : Einer deiner Freunde der Deutsch-Abteilung ruft dich an und erzählt dir eine Nachricht. Wie reagierst du

Freund Y

Y : Hallo mein(e) Freund(in),alles gut ?

Du: Ach! Super!

Y : Weißt du ? Ich habe gestern in der Zeitung gelesen, dass Homosexualität in der Elfenbeinküste bald legalisiert werden könnte.

Du: Humm!

Y : Ja, ich bin ein bisschen überrascht, aber ich finde es trotzdem toll !

Du: Bist du sicher?

Situation C : Dein bester Freund ruft dich an und informiert dich über die Ergebnisse der akademischen Prüfungen. Wie reagierst du darauf ?

Freund Z

Z : Hallo ! Du hast alle Prüfungen bestanden, ich auch.

Du: ich werde sehr glücklich sein

Situation A : Du sprichst mit deinem Freund, der nun in Deutschland lebt. Er kündigt dir seine Ankunft nach Heimat an. Wie reagierst du ?

X : Hallo ! Wie geht es dir ?

Du : Es geht mir sehr gut und du?

X : Mir geht es leider nicht gut.

Du : Warum ? was hat du ?

X : Meine Mutter ist gestern gestorben. Meine Schwester hat mir geschrieben.

Du : Ha lyako ,

X : Ich komme also bald zu Hause.

Du : Ich warte dich darauf .

X : Vielen Dank

Situation B : Einer deiner Freunde der Deutsch-Abteilung ruft dich an und erzählt dir eine Nachricht. Wie reagierst du

Freund Y

Y : Hallo mein(e) Freund(in),alles gut ?

Du : Ja, es geht mir gut .

Y : Weißt du ? Ich habe gestern in der Zeitung gelesen, dass Homosexualität in der Elfenbeinküste bald legalisiert werden könnte.

Du : Was ? wirklich es ist unmöglich .

Y : Ja, ich bin ein bisschen überrascht, aber ich finde es trotzdem toll !

Du : Was bin du Kopkoo, es ist unmöglich

Situation C : Dein bester Freund ruft dich an und informiert dich über die Ergebnisse der akademischen Prüfungen. Wie reagierst du darauf ?

Freund Z

Z : Hallo ! Du hast alle Prüfungen bestanden, ich auch.

Du : Ich bin sehr zufrieden, ich ein bisschen überrascht, weil es war schwierig

Situation A : Du sprichst mit deinem Freund, der nun in Deutschland lebt. Er kündigt dir seine Ankunft nach Heimat an. Wie reagierst du ?

X : Hallo ! Wie geht es dir ?

Du : ..es geht mir gut

X : Mir geht es leider nicht gut.

Du :..warum ?

X : Meine Mutter ist gestern gestorben. Meine Schwester hat mir geschrieben.

Du :..Oh!! schade

X : Ich komme also bald zu Hause.

Du :..OK

X : Vielen Dank .

Situation B : Einer deiner Freunde der Deutsch-Abteilung ruft dich an und erzählt dir eine Nachricht. Wie reagierst du

Freund Y

Y : Hallo mein(e) Freund(in),alles gut ?

Du :..ja..........

Y : Weißt du ? Ich habe gestern in der Zeitung gelesen, dass Homosexualität in der Elfenbeinküste bald legalisiert werden könnte.

Du :..das ist nicht gut

Y : Ja, ich bin ein bisschen überrascht, aber ich finde es trotzdem toll !

Du :...Hmmm !!!

Situation C : Dein bester Freund ruft dich an und informiert dich über die Ergebnisse der akademischen Prüfungen. Wie reagierst du darauf ?

Freund Z

Z : Hallo ! Du hast alle Prüfungen bestanden, ich auch.

Du :...~~[illegible]~~, waouuuu !!!

Situation A : Du sprichst mit deinem Freund, der nun in Deutschland lebt. Er kündigt dir seine Ankunft nach Heimat an. Wie reagierst du ?

X : Hallo ! Wie geht es dir ?

Du : Hallo! es geht mir gut. und du?

X : Mir geht es leider nicht gut.

Du : Hum! yacoi.

X : Meine Mutter ist gestern gestorben. Meine Schwester hat mir geschrieben.

Du : Beileid mein Freund.

X : Ich komme also bald zu Hause.

Du : ok, ich warte auf dir

X : Vielen Dank .

Situation B : Einer deiner Freunde der Deutsch-Abteilung ruft dich an und erzählt dir eine Nachricht. Wie reagierst du

Freund Y

Y : Hallo mein(e) Freund(in),alles gut ?

Du : Ja!

Y : Weißt du ? Ich habe gestern in der Zeitung gelesen, dass Homosexualität in der Elfenbeinküste bald legalisiert werden könnte.

Du : Ich bin überracht!.

Y : Ja, ich bin ein bisschen überrascht, aber ich finde es trotzdem toll !

Du : das ist nicht gut

Situation C : Dein bester Freund ruft dich an und informiert dich über die Ergebnisse der akademischen Prüfungen. Wie reagierst du darauf ?

Freund Z

Z : Hallo ! Du hast alle Prüfungen bestanden, ich auch.

Du : Vielen dank!.

Situation A : Du sprichst mit deinem Freund, der nun in Deutschland lebt. Er kündigt dir seine Ankunft nach Heimat an. Wie reagierst du ?

X : Hallo ! Wie geht es dir ?

Du : Es geht mir gut !

X : Mir geht es leider nicht gut.

Du : was ist los !

X : Meine Mutter ist gestern gestorben. Meine Schwester hat mir geschrieben.

Du : Haa Yako !

X : Ich komme also bald zu Hause.

Du : ok. Ich warte dich auf!

X : Vielen Dank .

Situation B : Einer deiner Freunde der Deutsch-Abteilung ruft dich an und erzählt dir eine Nachricht. Wie reagierst du

Freund Y

Y : Hallo mein(e) Freund(in),alles gut ?

Du : ja... Alles ist Gut bei mir!

Y : Weißt du ? Ich habe gestern in der Zeitung gelesen, dass Homosexualität in der Elfenbeinküste bald legalisiert werden könnte.

Du : wirklich !

Y : Ja, ich bin ein bisschen überrascht, aber ich finde es trotzdem toll !

Du : nicht für mich!

Situation C : Dein bester Freund ruft dich an und informiert dich über die Ergebnisse der akademischen Prüfungen. Wie reagierst du darauf ?

Freund Z

Z : Hallo ! Du hast alle Prüfungen bestanden, ich auch.

Du : Ach so! Ich bin sehr zufrieden darüber !

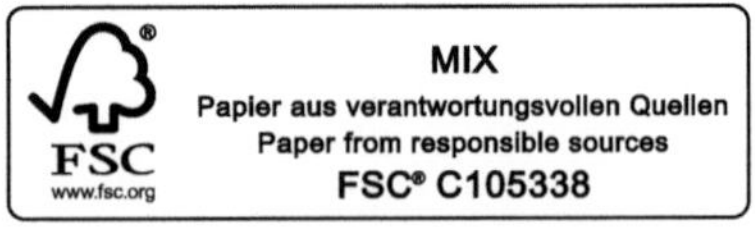

Printed by Books on Demand GmbH, Norderstedt / Germany